BREAKFAST SMOOTHIE FOR WEIGHT LOSS:

Delicious Breakfast Smoothies to Jumpstart Your Weight Loss.

Saint Dowell

TABLE OF CONTENTS

INTRODUCTION

You have to answer the dreaded query "What's for breakfast?" each morning.

To eat healthily, you must ensure that you get enough fiber, vegetables, and protein to start the day off properly while monitoring your calorie intake. Enter ideas for nutritious smoothies.

According to **Julie Andrews**, RDN, the creator of The **Healthy Epicurean**, nutritious well-balanced smoothies can be a great addition to a well-balanced diet for weight reduction and general health.

However, not just any smoothie would do because, as she points out, some may contain a lot more sugar and calories but fewer nutrients that aid in weight reduction and general health.

If you drink protein-rich breakfast smoothies, you won't likely feel famished until after noon, advises **Keri Gans,** RDN, author of The Small Change Diet. Additionally, "for satiety as well as overall nutrition, a little fat and fiber are needed."

Any kind of berry, banana, spinach, kale, avocado, low-fat basic Greek yogurt, low-fat milk, a non-dairy milk substitute with protein, chia seeds, flax seeds, hemp seeds, and nut butter are all excellent additions to smoothies, according to **Gans.**

According to **Leah Johnston,** RDN, a culinary nutritionist, if you want to prepare ahead of time, consider freezing the majority of the ingredients for your smoothies (such as fruits, seeds, and vegetables) in individual bags and taking one out as required each day.

Smoothies have been popular among consumers who are concerned about their health, and we must confess that they are wonderfully easy to make, filled with fruits and vegetables, and readily available in a matter of seconds.

However, not every smoothie is made equal. In actuality, a lot of store-bought milkshakes are overly sweet and caloric. Therefore, if you're looking for healthy smoothie recipes, we have the ingredients, blend-ready tips, and blend-ready techniques for you.

How to make a nutritious milkshake, If you have a good mix of ingredients and nutrients, such as protein, carbohydrates, and healthy fats, smoothies can make a nutritious breakfast.

This book states that smoothies can be a convenient and healthy way to include several nutrients to help jump-start your day.

Mathis particularly appreciates that smoothies can be tailored to any flavor or preference. She stresses the significance of making informed substitutions to guarantee that you're receiving all the nutrients your body requires. For instance, protein powder adds a powerful punch of the macronutrient to smoothies, but Mathis also enjoys almonds, cottage cheese, chia seeds, and other foods that are rich in protein.

A source of healthy fat, such as nuts or avocado, as well as additional fiber from vegetables, flax seeds, hemp seeds, or chia seeds, can also aid in supplying necessary vitamins, minerals, and antioxidants, according to the expert.

Give me my crown and scepter, and I will rule the land of good ideals. I'm frequently enticed by a wide range of lofty objectives (run a marathon! take more vitamins! create my yogurt!). Why not start modestly, like having a healthy breakfast or snack, rather than worrying about too many grand goals? Let's guzzle down more healthy breakfast smoothies and declare victory!

I'm sharing this collection of nutritious breakfast smoothies that are stuffed with all the protein, fruits, and vegetables you need to power through our healthy, realistic objectives. the day.

I'm offering this collection of healthful morning smoothies that are jam-packed with all the protein, fruits, and vegetables you need to power your day o fuel your healthy, realistic objectives.

Eating healthy is enjoyable and not a bother when the meals are as delicious as these.

You'll know how much I adore healthy smoothies if you've ever visited the smoothie section of my website. Despite having excellent nutritional value, they taste like a treat.

Extra points for being so simple to prepare in advance.

So let's start each day with little steps, delicious breakfast smoothies, and a nourishing breakfast. Cheers!

CHAPTER ONE

IS HAVING A SMOOTHIE FOR BREAKFAST HEALTHY?

Smoothies can be a very wholesome breakfast option; the trick is to choose high-quality ingredients and consume them in moderation.
When these recommendations are followed, having a smoothie for breakfast each day is appropriate.

Smoothies for breakfast that are incredibly healthy and delicious are quick and simple to create.

To help you feel fuller for longer, seek a nutritious breakfast smoothie that is low in sugar and high in protein, fiber, and healthy fats.

CHAPTER TWO

WHAT GOES INTO A SMOOTHIE?

There are so many different ingredients that may be included in a breakfast smoothie.

Different advantageous effects are provided by each group of substances. Some of my favorite suggestions for things to include in your morning smoothie are listed below:

Suitable fats.

Chia seeds, coconut milk, or the nut butter of your choice. As a result, the smoothie is more satiating and filling between meals. Be mindful of quantities; typically add around 1 tablespoon.

Fiber and protein additions.

Greek yogurt or your preferred protein powder is a quick and simple recipe.

Fruit.

Fruit smoothies for breakfast are a perennial
favorite. My favorites are blueberries and
strawberries.

Smoothies are naturally sweetened by
bananas.
Green food tastes can be covered up with
mango and pineapple.
Fruits that you wouldn't expect, like apples
or melons, can also be delicious.
Vegetables. Smoothies can include spinach,
kale, avocado, carrots, and even beets.

Taste Enhancements.

Dates, vanilla, cinnamon, honey, maple
syrup, and all of these are great methods to
enhance the flavor of your smoothie.
Liquid.

My preferred almond milk for smoothies is unsweetened. You can also use coconut water, a different sort of milk, juice, plain water, or even juice in moderation as it is high in sugar but low in fiber.

CHAPTER THREE

DO MORNING SMOOTHIES HELP WITH WEIGHT LOSS?

Smoothies for breakfast that are filling, high in protein, and low in calories can help you lose weight.

Choosing hefty breakfast smoothies will ensure that you are not ravenous by mid-morning.

For recipe inspiration, check out the Healthy Breakfast Smoothies for Weight Loss category below.
The above is meant as a general recommendation. Please get in touch with a nutritionist or your doctor for more details or particular dietary advice for you.

CHAPTER FOUR

HOW TO PREPARE AND PRESERVE SMOOTHIES.

The majority of smoothies may be prepared the night before and kept in the refrigerator.

 Smoothies can be kept in the fridge for up to a day.

- The smoothie should be put in an airtight container since the less air that touches it, the better.

- Before serving, stir, and make it in advance.

- Make the smoothie as suggested, then transfer to an airtight mason jar that is freezer-safe and freeze it for up to three months.

- The dish should thaw overnight in the refrigerator before being served.

CHAPTER FIVE

EQUIPMENT TO MAKE SMOOTHIE.

Blender.

Blenders are powerful equipment that makes everything incredibly smooth and creamy.
This less expensive approach using a blender is still excellent, but you might need to add extra liquid or add the frozen fruit more gradually.

Straws made of stainless steel.

Anything you drink via these stainless steel straws tastes incredibly refreshing. So that I won't have to ask for a plastic or paper straw when I'm out, I try to keep some in my purse. These work wonderfully for bringing smoothies with you.
Dark Cup.

A terrific technique to prepare (hide) green smoothies for kids' breakfast.

But, considering that nutritionists advise against drinking food to feel full, it's generally best to stick to one smoothie per day and eat regular meals and snacks throughout the day.
Include at least 25 grams of protein in your smoothie if you want to use it as a meal, and at least 10 grams of protein if you want to use it as a snack.

With their nutrient-dense fruit and vegetable blends, creamy milk, protein, probiotic-rich yogurt, and other healthy ingredients, these tasty, healthy smoothies make eating well simpler.
Just a heads up: If you're trying to reduce added sugar in your diet, you can omit the fruit juice or honey that some of these recipes call for increased wetness.

CHAPTER SIX

SMOOTHIE RECIPES FOR WEIGHT LOSS.

A fruit smoothie bowl.

Who said that smoothie could only be sipped?

- Blend frozen blueberries, almond butter, vanilla, and almond milk until deliciously smooth.

- Garnish the mixture with hemp and fresh blueberries after dividing it into two halves.

- To make the breakfast bowl of your dreams, add blueberries, hemp seeds, vanilla granola, and more.

The Berry, Chia, and Mint Smoothie.

Our preferred shade of red is found in this smoothie, which also includes strawberries, raspberries, and beets.
It offers a good deal of gastrointestinal-friendly fiber and a cool sip thanks to the surprise addition of mint.

Green pineapple and coconut-flavored smoothie.

The exotic flavors of pineapple, coconut, banana, and lime are given a healthful boost by the inclusion of baby spinach.
It is a filling cup that will make any time of day seem like an island getaway.

Smoothie for Stress Relief.

When combined with raspberries, hemp seeds, and a peach, tangy kefir's stress-relieving qualities may be enhanced.
But, if you are unable to find hemp seeds, substitute a spoonful of almond butter,

which also boosts magnesium levels, which is crucial for lowering stress.

Smoothie with kale and cream.

This smoothie may be found in the Smoothies & Juices section under Balanced Gut on the Prevention website. Greek yogurt is a natural method to get more protein and probiotics to enhance gut health.

- A blender should be used to incorporate 1 cup of roughly chopped kale, and 1 1/2 cups of frozen pineapple chunks.

- 1/2 cup of plain Greek yogurt, 1/2 cup of unsweetened almond milk, and 1 teaspoon of honey.

- The mixture should be stirred until it foams and becomes smooth.

Orange-Pineapple Smoothie Bowl.

This smoothie bowl is a delicious way to mix up your diet.
Greek yogurt, heart-healthy cashews, and citrus fruit, which are strong in vitamin C, are all included.

- A blend of 1/2 cup fat-free Greek yogurt.

- 1/2 cup frozen pineapple chunks, 1/4 teaspoon vanilla extract.

- 1/2 navel orange and 1/2 ruby grapefruit are made.

- After churning the ingredients until it is smooth, divide them into 2 bowls.

- On top, incorporate more orange and grapefruit, chia seeds, unsweetened coconut flakes, and finely chopped cashews.

Peach Blueberry Smoothie.

Even though it's January, this delicious concoction's peaches and blueberries will make you feel like it's summertime. Moreover, nutrient-dense kale will assist you in getting your recommended daily intake of vegetables. A sprinkle of cinnamon is the perfect finishing ingredient.

- A handful of kale, and four slices of fresh or frozen peaches (about 1/2 cup).

- 1/4 cup of blueberries and 1/4 teaspoon of ground cinnamon are blended with 1 cup of chilled almond or vanilla soy milk.

- Blend after smoothing.

Banana-blueberry-soy smoothie.

Succulent blueberries burst with flavor in this nutritious smoothie, which is also packed with potassium-rich banana and vanilla for sweetness.

- Blend 1 1/4 cups light soy milk with 1/2 cup frozen blueberries.

- 1/2 cup frozen banana, and 1/8 teaspoon pure vanilla extract.

- Blend for 20 to 30 seconds until smooth. You can increase the amount of milk by up to 1/4 cup if you like a thinner consistency.

Oat-based Peaches and Cream Smoothie.

Insufficient time to enjoy a leisurely meal? Try this breakfast porridge that is packed with probiotics. Whole-grain oats include prebiotic fiber that promotes digestive health.

This Smoothies & Juices from Prevention recipe yields two smoothies:

Blend 1/2 cup whole milk,1/2 cup Greek yogurt, 1/2 cup rolled oats, 1/2 cup frozen banana, and 1 cup frozen peaches until smooth.

Pineapple Passion Smoothie.

Your need for an ice cream cone will be sated by this decadently thick smoothie recipe.
In addition, pineapple contains bromelain, an enzyme that helps break down protein and may reduce bloating.

- Combine 6 ice cubes, 1 cup of diced pineapple, and 1 cup of low-fat or light vanilla yogurt.

- To produce a smooth consistency, mix all the ingredients and pulse as necessary.

Smoothie with milk and honey.

Use the celery in your produce drawer with this juice that has been pureed.

it with grapes, cucumber, and almond milk for a refreshing snack.

- 1 1/2 cups unsweetened almond milk, 1 medium Kirby cucumber, 1 cup seedless green grapes, 2 medium stalks celery, and 1 Tbsp honey should be blended.

- Mix until smooth; yield two servings.

Smoothie for Silky Skin.

You'll love how your skin responds to this beverage from Prevention's Smoothies and Juices!
Beta-carotene, an antioxidant that the body transforms into vitamin A, is abundant in apricots and carrots.

The vitamin may be able to counteract skin aging, UV ray damage, and pollution-related skin damage.

- Blend 1/4 cup grated carrot, 1/2 cup whole milk Greek yogurt, 1 tablespoon honey, 1/2 tablespoon cinnamon, 2 chopped dried apricots, and 1 fresh apricot in a blender (pitted and coarsely chopped).

- Once smooth, blend.

Lean, Mean, Green Machine.

This smoothie is the perfect post-workout recovery beverage.
Coconut water aids in rehydration, sweet banana and kiwi supply potassium and vitamin C, and protein powder helps replace the calories you expended.

- 1 medium banana, 1 kiwi, 1 cup unsweetened almond milk, 1 cup spinach, 1 scoop vanilla whey protein powder, and 1/2 cup coconut water should all be in a blender.

- blended in creamy and blend-dreamy.

Berry-Banana-Oat Smoothie.

Smoothies with oats have more body, and the resistant starch in oats, a whole grain, keeps you satiated for longer.

An additional benefit of resistant starch? Compared to other fibers, it produces less gas.

- Blend 1 cup vanilla low-fat yogurt, 2 cups frozen strawberries, 1 banana, 1/2 cup rolled oats, 1/2 cup orange juice, and 1 Tbsp, honey.

- Pour the mixture into a blender and blend.

Caribbean Dream Smoothie.

If you frequently get queasy before important events, try drinking this smoothie from Prevention's Smoothies & Juices.

It includes banana, which has magnesium, a calming mineral; also, the bacteria in the yogurt may reduce anxiety.

- Blend Smoothly combine 1/2 cup pineapple chunks, 1/4 cup 2% Greek yogurt, 1/4 cup chilled unsweetened coconut milk, 1/4 cup orange juice, and 1/4 large banana.

- Sip it two hours before you need to relax your nerves for the finest results in reducing anxiety.

Smoothie with green ginger.

The delightful shade of green in this smoothie is a result of the combination of baby spinach and Granny Smith apples. Healthy lipids and plant protein are added by hemp seeds.

- Combine 2 cups of baby spinach that has been packed, 1 Granny Smith apple that has been chopped, 3/4 cup of coconut water, 1/4 cup of lemon juice, 2 Tbsp. of hemp seeds, 3 Tbsp.

of minced ginger, 1 Tbsp. of raw honey, and 1 12 cups of ice cubes.

- Once smooth, blend. The dish serves two.

Cranberry Banana Smoothie.

The highlight of this satiating, fiber-rich delight is the autumn berry. The banana adds bulk and sweetness, the almond milk keeps the calorie count low, and the maple syrup gives it a hint of seasonal sweetness.

- Blend 1 banana, 1 cup unsweetened almond milk, 1 cup frozen cranberries, 1 tablespoon maple syrup, and 1/2 cup ice cubes.

- Mix until foamy and well-combine.

Apple Crisp Smoothie.

Enjoy this delectable smoothie that features sweet apple cider, Greek yogurt, oats, almonds, and comforting spices to capture the flavor of autumn.

Moreover, it contains a lot of protein and the fiber beta-glucan, which increases endurance.

Smoothie with green tea, blueberries, and bananas.

Simply zap 3 Tbsp. of water in a bowl in the microwave for a few seconds to make this smoothie with antioxidant-rich green tea.

- Add 1 green tea bag after that, and let it steep for 3 minutes.

- After removing the tea bag, whisk in 2 teaspoons of honey until it dissolves.

- Blend 1 1/2 cups frozen blueberries, a medium banana, and 3/4 cups light vanilla soy milk with calcium fortification in a blender.

- When all ingredients are blended, add the tea.

Mocha protein shake.

This popular breakfast has a milkshake-like flavor.

The key component? Walnuts.

These nuts are rich in protein and heart-healthy omega-3 fatty acids, which are proven to reduce inflammation and safeguard the cardiovascular system. The dosage This smoothie is ideal for the morning when combined with some black coffee.

- Blend 1 1/2 cups of pre-made, cooled black coffee with 1 cup of ice cubes, 1/4 cup of walnuts, 1 heaping tablespoon of unsweetened cocoa powder, and 6 tablespoons of chocolate protein powder.

- Once smooth, blend.

- This dish serves two people.

Powerful Pumpkin Smoothie.

This smoothie has Greek yogurt for a creamy, protein-rich foundation.
In addition to the pure skin, all sweetness is added with maple syrup and pumpkin pie spice.

- Blend 1/4 avocado, 2 tablespoons of ground flaxseed, 1 tablespoon of maple syrup, and 1/2 tsp.

- pumpkin pie spice, and 1/2 cup pure canned pumpkin that has been frozen in an ice cube tray. until creamy, blend.

Strawberry-Kiwi Smoothie.

Use organic kiwis for this tasty, low-calorie smoothie recipe to make it healthier because they have higher levels of heart-healthy polyphenols and vitamin C.

- 1 Blend 1 1/2 tablespoons of honey, 1 ripe banana, 1 kiwi, 5 frozen strawberries, and 1 1/4 cups of cool apple juice until smooth, and pure.

Tropical Papaya Perfection Smoothie.

This milkshake-like breakfast smoothie with coconut flavoring is delicious. You'll be transported to a tropical island with only one drink.

- One papaya, cut into chunks.

- one cup of fat-free plain yogurt, one teaspoon of coconut extract, half a cup of fresh pineapple chunks, half a cup of crushed ice, and one teaspoon of ground flaxseed.

- blend The mixture should be smooth and icy after around 30 seconds of processing.

Banana Almond Protein Smoothie.

After a strenuous workout, coconut water helps replenish electrolytes while creamy almond butter provides healthy fats.

The protein content is kept high with Greek yogurt and a scoop of whey.

- Add 1 frozen banana, 1 cup of juice, and 3 Tbsp. almond butter, 1 scoop whey protein powder, 1/2 cup plain

Greek yogurt, 1/2 cup coconut water, and 1/2 cup hemp seeds to a blender.

- Blend until smooth.

- The dish serves two.

Berry Good Workout Smoothie.

With this quick and simple smoothie recipe, you may quickly get the energy you need to get through your workout.
Add a teaspoon of organic kale powder for a calcium boost.

- Add 1/2 cup ice cubes, 1 1/2 cups sliced strawberries, 1 cup blueberries, 1/2 cup raspberries, 2 tablespoons honey, and 1 teaspoon fresh lemon juice.

- Once smooth, blend.

Tutti-Frutti Smoothie.

This nutritious and energizing snack is citrus-infused thanks to a dash of orange juice.

- Just half a cup of mixed frozen berries, half a cup of canned crushed pineapple in juice, half a cup of plain yogurt, half a cup of sliced ripe bananas, and half a cup of orange juice are required.

- When smooth, the process lasts roughly two minutes. The dish serves two.

- (To reduce the amount of sugar, substitute fresh pineapple for canned pineapple and orange juice.)

Mango Crazy Smoothie.

Take advantage of the ripe mango's capacity to ward off disease with this delectable smoothie recipe.

- First, combine 1 cup of fat-free frozen vanilla yogurt, 1 can of pineapple chunks packed with juice, 1 large mango that has been peeled and pitted, and 1 ripe banana in a blender.

- Once smooth, blend.

- then gradually add roughly a cup of ice.

Berry Avocado Antioxidant Smoothie.

This smoothie recipe, which is loaded with vitamins, minerals, and antioxidants, relies on frozen avocado to give it a rich, creamy texture.

Moreover, a blend of antioxidant-rich frozen berries, flax seeds, and spinach.

Smoothie with Yellow Fruit and Turmeric.

A well-known superfood with anti-inflammatory and antioxidant effects is turmeric.

One of the spice's main ingredients, curcumin, may aid improve cognition, reduce joint discomfort, reduce the risk of developing certain malignancies, and diminish the signs of depression.
Why are you holding out? Create this smoothie, which is brimming with it.

Smoothie with peanut butter and jelly.

This is a smoothie recipe that will bring back memories of your favorite childhood treat.

This smoothie's sweet and salty flavor comes from a combination of berries and peanut butter powder.
Also, the vanilla powder gives you endurance, preventing you from being hungry an hour after consuming this rich beverage.

Pumpkin Coconut Smoothie.

You may feel good about consuming this thick and creamy smoothie because there is no added sugar.
Also, it simply requires five ingredients and five minutes to cook.
Also, it complies with a variety of diets, including vegan, vegetarian, gluten-free, and Paleo.
For more protein, think about including a scoop of collagen powder.

Green Smoothie for Detox with Chia Seeds.

Here's a fantastic chance to try chia seeds if you haven't already. These little but strong seeds are a fantastic source of heart-healthy omega-3 fatty acids. Because of their plant protein strength, they also help you feel filled for longer.

The ideal breakfast treat is this delicious concoction of spinach, unsweetened almond milk, frozen pineapple, and naturally sweet banana.

Overnight Oatmeal Smoothie with Caramel Apple.

For chilly mornings when you're seeking a fall treat, try this vegan, gluten-free breakfast smoothie.

Don't panic; this recipe does not contain caramel.

Instead, this blogger substitutes dates, which also provide natural sweetness and provide minerals, fiber, and antioxidants. Together with fiber and protein, rolled oats also contain apples and cinnamon.

deliver that indubitably comforting flavor.

You may save so much time in the mornings by putting this enticing concoction in the refrigerator the night before.

 Smoothie with carrot cake.

Although carrots aren't often the highlight of a breakfast smoothie, this creamy concoction will change your mind.
The banana slices, sliced pineapple, walnuts, cinnamon, and nutmeg blend flawlessly with the carrots to create a smoothie that tastes exactly like a slice of carrot cake.

Cranberry Citrus Smoothie.

This delightful citrus beverage delivers a shot of vitamin C and a tangy, reviving flavor from a combination of cranberries and oranges.
A base of plain Greek yogurt adds extra protein and richness, while frozen bananas

and a splash of vanilla flavor provide
balance.
Oranges can be used in place of any other
citrus fruits, so feel free to substitute
tangerines or clementines if you prefer.

CHAPTER SEVEN

MAKING A HEALTHFUL SMOOTHIE.

According to **Johnston**, if you don't pay attention to the balance of macronutrients in the components, smoothies can quickly become carb-heavy.

She advises categorizing the ingredients you add to smoothies in the following sequence.

Protein. Greek yogurts, kefir, nut butter, cottage cheese, dairy- or plant-based milk, as well as casein, hemp, pea, and whey protein powders.

Veggies. Dark leafy greens like kale or spinach, cucumber, and cooked beets and carrots.

wholesome fats. Fish oil, nut butter, avocado, avocado oil, and extra virgin olive oil.

Fruits. Bananas, berries, pineapple, and acai.

Additional carbohydrates. whole grains like quinoa or oats.

Additional nutrition. Matcha, turmeric, ginger, hemp seeds, chia seeds, cacao, and flaxseed.

Liquid. Coconut water, milk made from animals or plants, or ordinary water.

Although some ingredients may fit into more than one category, doing so guarantees that your smoothie is a balanced meal.

Honey or maple syrup can be used to offer a little more sweetness, but **Johnston** advises against using too much or items with a lot of added sugar, such as flavored yogurts or juices.

Although they might give your smoothie a gritty feel, nuts are another excellent source of healthy fats.

Use soft foods alone, and avoid employing too-hard foods.
The blender is not being intentionally harmed in this smoothie-making process, claims Johnston. Raw beets or carrots could be too tough for a typical blender to handle, so cook them first by roasting or steaming them.

CHAPTER EIGHT

CAN YOU HAVE A SMOOTHIE EVERY DAY?

According to **Johnston**, it is quite OK to substitute a nutritious and well-balanced smoothie for breakfast each day.
You are consuming all of these items at once as opposed to eating them separately. even more, nourishment than you would from other sources.

from a typical breakfast item like cereal or a bagel.

However, Johnston advises experimenting with the recipe by adding more protein, fiber (like oats), or healthy fat to boost the smoothie's satiating ability if you start substituting your breakfast with one and discover that it isn't as satisfying as your usual food.

CONCLUSION

Smoothies are common lunch and snack options that may be customized to almost any taste or dietary requirement.

Its nutritional value is greatly influenced by its ingredients.

The most nutrient-dense smoothies are those made with whole foods such as fruits, vegetables, yogurt, and healthy fats.

In contrast, smoothies with a lot of added sugar are less nutrient-dense and may have long-term negative effects on health.

Protein and fiber-rich smoothies may even help you lose weight by keeping you satisfied.

If you're looking for a creative way to improve the number of fruits and veggies in your diet, smoothies might be the way to go.